Essential Oils 2017:

30 Amazing Essential Oil Recipes for Diffusers

Table of content

30 Amazing Essential Oil Recipes for Diffusers 1

Introduction 4

Chapter 1 – Amazing Essential Oil Diffusers for Sleep 6

Essential Oils for Loneliness 9

Chapter 2 – Get Rid of Stress and Anxiety with Essential Oil Diffusers....11

Chapter 3 – Essential Oil Diffusers to Enhance Happiness 19

Bergamot Essential Oil..19

Geranium Essential Oil 20

Chapter 4 – Essential Oil Diffusers to Manage Anger...........................22

Peace and Calming Blend...22

Ylang Ylang...22

Roman Chamomile Essential Oil 23

Lavender Essential Oil 23

Geranium Essential Oil 24

Sandalwood Essential Oil..24

Blue Tansy Essential Oil..25

Tips to Diffuse Your Blend 27

Diffuser 28

Chapter 5 – Increase Your Confidence with Essential Oil Diffusers 29

Cypress Essential Oil 29

Peppermint Essential Oils 29

Sandalwood Essential Oil..30

Bergamot Essential Oil..30

Rosemary Essential Oil 31

Tea Tree Essential Oil..31

Chamomile Essential Oil..31

Ylang-Ylang Essential Oil 32

Diffuser to Increase Your Alertness..32

Precautionary Tips for Essential Oil..34

Conclusion 38

FREE Bonus Reminder 39

Introduction

It is really enjoyable to use essential oil blends in a diffuser and enjoy the benefits of aromatherapy. You can add a few drops of essential oils in a diffuser to get the advantage of therapeutic aromatherapy. There are different types of diffusers that you can choose from candle burners to lamp rings and water vapor diffusers. Heat may cause essential oils to degrade and evaporate quickly, and cold air diffusers should be preferred over heat diffusers. You can use different blends of diffusers together to create soothing effects and enjoy their health effects.

The essential oils work in a particular way because whenever you inhale an essential oil, the molecules of its odor may travel up to the nose allied to the nerves of the olfactory membranes in the nose. These molecules can excite the inside layer of nerve cells and enhance the electrical impulses to the olfactory bulb of your brain. This particular part of your brain transmits the impulses to the amygdala. The amygdala is the place where the memories are usually stored, and connected to the limbic system of the brain.

There is a direct connection between the limbic system and the other parts of your brain. These parts of your brain are responsible for controlling the heart rate, breathing, blood pressure, memory, stress level and hormones. The aroma of essential oils can excite the release of hormones and alter the behavior of your body and mind. The fragrance and unique molecular structure of the essential oils can stimulate the limbic lobe. You can inhale essential oils to reduce stress and emotional shock. You can trigger the production of thyroid hormones and other important hormones to improve your health and increase your life.

Emotional Brain Give Response to Smell Only

Amygdala is an important part of the brain that plays a significant role in treating emotional shocks. The scents of essential oils directly linked to the emotional states and behavior of a person. Smell is one of the five senses with a direct connection to the emotional control center. It can gradually overcome the fear, anger, anxiety, depression and all negative emotions.

You can learn about calming blends to promote your sleep, reduce stress and anxiety and enhance your mood. This book has lots of things for you to discover.

Chapter 1 – Amazing Essential Oil Diffusers for Sleep

There are lots of essential oils that can help you to relieve the symptoms of stress, anxiety and depression and enjoy a sound sleep. You can treat your anxiety with the use of some scented essential oils. A right scent will make you happy; therefore, you should select a scent carefully. Following are some essential oils that can help you to get rid of tension and depression:

- **Basil Essential Oil:** It can enhance your mood and work to remove emotions of anxiety, fatigue and depress.

- **Clary Safe Essential Oil:** It is an excellent essential oil to get rid of insomnia, tension, anxiety, and depression.

- **Frankincense:** If you are suffering from stress, anxiety, fear and tension, then you should use this essential oil to slow down these emotions.

- **Geranium Essential Oil:** It may reduce your stress and depression because it naturally works to enhance the spirit and release the negative emotions out.

- **Jasmine Essential Oil:** It is a relaxing and an antispasmodic essential oil with mood-lifting properties.

- **Lemon Essential Oil:** The refreshing scent of the lemon essential oil can enhance your mood. It enables you to fight with the stress, negative emotions, and depression.

- **Mandarin Essential Oil:** The antispasmodic properties help you to uplift the spirit.

- **Marjoram:** If you are feeling grief, fear, rejection, anxiety, and loneliness, then this is an excellent essential oil to enhance your mood.

- **Wild Orange:** It is good to increase your energy and enhance your mood. It is excellent to relieve the feelings of anger, irritation, and nervousness.

- **Palmarosa:** It is excellent for the treatment of nervous tension and anxiety.

- **Rose:** It can stimulate the sense of well-being by treating tension and nervousness.

- **Roman Chamomile:** It is ideal to relax your body and mind. It is an ultimate treatment for the depression and stress.

- **Sandalwood:** Its scent has magical properties to relieve tension and stress.

- **Ylang-Ylang:** The relaxing scent of ylang-ylang is equally good to energize both men and women. The scent of this essential oil can increase your confidence and treat depression, insomnia, and stress.

BLENDS *for sleep!*

6 Drops Rutavala

4 Drops Lavender
4 Drops Peace & Calming

4 Drops Lavender
3 Drops Bergamot

4 Drops Frankincense
3 Drops Vetiver

2 Drops Lavender
2 Drops Cedarwood
2 Drops Peace & Calming

3 Drops Lavender
3 Drops Roman Chamomile
1 Drop Vetiver

2 Drops Lavender
2 Drops Vetiver
2 Drops Valerian
2 Drops Orange

4 Drops Lavender
1 Drop Bergamot
1 Drop Patchouli
1 Drop Ylang Ylang

Essential Oils for Loneliness

Isolation and loneliness are not good for anyone because it can harm you because during isolation, your mind filled with lots of negative thoughts and emotions. You prefer to live in isolation, but during the adverse times, it is important to take the help of your friends and love. The Ayurveda offers the best solution and it is meditation. You can talk to God during medication and offer a small prayer to comfort yourself. This will bring a great difference in your condition. There are some essential oils that will give you the energy to fight with the loneliness and support your mind.

Special Blend for Loneliness

If you are feeling lonely, then try this blend to get power for your mind and body:

- Rose oil

- Chamomile oil

- Frankincense oil

- Clary sages oil

- Bergamot oil

Take 1 to 2 drops of the oils and add into your bathtub to take a bath. You need to use a diffuser to reduce the intensity of the oils. You can use olive oil or almond oil as a carrier oil to defuse the blend. It will be good to apply this blend on your handkerchief and keep it with you to get energy and power to fight lonesomeness.

Note: The helichrysum and palo santo essential oils are also good to treat loneliness.

Chapter 2 – Get Rid of Stress and Anxiety with Essential Oil Diffusers

If you are dealing with anxious feelings, then it is important to use essential oils because these are better to use as compared to medicines. Following are some essential oils that you can use to treat your anxiety:

Balance Essential Oil

This essential oil is a blend of rosewood, blue tansy, spruce, and frankincense. It is an ideal essential oil to treat your anxiety. You can get a feeling of calmness with the use of this oil. It is a natural remedy used to calm down your nerves and promote the relaxation. The chamomile is used to soothe your nerves. The Frankincense can promote your relaxation and relieve the feelings of sorrow.

Lavender Essential Oil

If you are dealing with anxiousness, then you can try the lavender essential oil. Its scent is really calm and attractive, and you can use it in the water while taking a bath. You can also add it few drops in the deodorant to make it relaxing. There is a number of scientific proves that the lavender can reduce the anxiety and enhance the mood of patients.

Wild Orange Essential Oils

Wild orange essential oil is a great choice to reduce anxiety and boost your mood. It can increase your happiness and well-being. It is not good to eat any essential oil, but you can add a few drops of orange essential oils in your recipe to enhance citrus flavor.

Serenity Essential Oil

Serenity is a useful essential oil prepared to treat your anxiety. You can combine this essential oil with the lavender, sweet marjoram, ylang-ylang, sandalwood, and vanilla. These all oils have excellent properties, and you can enjoy a massage of these oils to promote sleep. The ylang-ylang is really beneficial for your central nervous system. The serenity can be applied topically or you may diffuse it in the air. You can apply it to the bottom of your feet before going to bed to enjoy a deep and relaxing sleep.

Bergamot Essential Oil

The bergamot is used to relieve the tension and stress, and it can also be used to improve the health of your skin. It features citrus scent and you can use it to enhance your mood. The bergamot can promote the relaxation by reducing the feelings of anxiousness. It is the best essential oil to apply to the skin or diffuse in the air to treating the tension and promote a good sleep. In order to enhance the benefits of essential oils, it will be good to use magnesium supplement to overcome your anxious feelings.

Grounding Blend

It is a useful blend of howood, spruce, frankincense and chamomile. If you are suffering from anxiety and tension, then this blend will really help you. It can promote the feelings of calmness and reduce your stress.

Application:

The grounding blend can be applied to your feet on a regular basis. You can also massage it over the back of your neck, heart and the wrists get better results.

Apply on the wrists and rub them together and inhale. You can mix this oil with a calming blend to increase its benefits.

Respiratory Blend

It is a versatile blend used for all respiratory issues. It is a combination of peppermint, lemon, ravensara lead, melaleuca and Cardamom seeds. It will help you to calm down your brain during anxiety.

Application:

Apply a few drops on your chest to relax your nerves and open your airways for relaxed breathing.

Frankincense

It is a king of essential oils that is why it is really valuable to slow down the fear, anxiety and tension. If you are suffering from stressful feelings, then it is an excellent choice for you. It can help you to combat the feelings of fear and anxiety.

Directions:

It is a great oil for regular use because it can promote your cellular balance. It can reduce feelings of anxiety, so use it in the diffuse state. You can inhale it, or massage your feet and back with a few drops of oil. Blend of lavender oil and wild orange can help you to get rid of anxiety.

Try a Joyful Blend

The smell of this oil will be great to treat the feelings of anxiety and tensions. It can treat anxiety and depression at the same time. The blend contains lavender, tangerine, elemi, lemon, Melissa, ylang-ylang, sandalwood, and osmanthus.

Directions:

You can apply it on your heart, bones, behind the ear, neck, forehead and wrists to reduce stress. Its regular application will help you to calm your mind and get rid of tensions.

Lemon Essential Oil

It is a versatile oil with lots of benefits because of its properties. The lemon oil is excellent to uplift your mood, revive your stressful feelings, and stimulate your feelings. The lemon enhances the sense of security and trust. It can help you to remove confusions and tensions. It can clear the obstacles and improve your feelings.

Directions:

You can use it on a regular basis in water. Just add 1 drop of essential oil in a glass of water and then use it for the whole day.

Calming Blend

If you want to promote relaxed feelings, then this blend is excellent for you. It can control your anger and promote good health with calmness. The blend contains sweet marjoram, lavender, ylang-ylang, roman chamomile, sandalwood, and vanilla bean.

Direction:

Use almost 5 drops of this blend in the hot water for relaxation. You can also apply it on the back of your neck and inhale it through a diffuser. Some drops should be applied to the bottoms of your feet before going to sleep. Awesome smell can leave excellent effects on your nerves.

Patchouli Essential Oil

It is a special oil to harmonize your mind and keep it stable without any tension. It can reduce the negative thoughts by relieving the depression and increase the joy in your life. You can recover from tension, stress and tiredness of mind.

Direction:

You can apply a diffused form of this oil to the base of your skull. Inhale the aroma of the oil to calm your fortitude and reduce disorganized thoughts.

Woody Diffuser for Calming Effects

Cypress oil: 2 drops

White first oil: 2 drops

Wintergreen oil: 2 drops

Spiced Chai

Cardamom oil: 3 drops

Cassia oil: 2 drops

Clove oil: 2 drops

Ginger oil: 1 drop

Enjoy Autumn Smell

Wild orange oil: 3 drops

Cinnamon bark oil: 2 drops

Clove oil: 1 drop

Calming Effects

Frankincense oil: 3 drops

White fir oil: 2 drops

Cedarwood oil: 1 drop

Boost Immunity

Rosemary oil: 1 drop

Clove oil: 1 drop

Cinnamon bark oil: 1 drop

Eucalyptus oil: 1 drop

Wild orange oil: 1 drop

Stress Buster Blend

Frankincense oil: 2 drops

Bergamot oil: 2 drops

Enhance Sleep

Lavender oil: 2 drops

Chamomile oil: 2 drops

Vetiver essential oil: 2 drops

Chapter 3 – Essential Oil Diffusers to Enhance Happiness

Everyone has its own reasons to become happy, but if you want to increase your joy, then you should use some essential oils. These oils can help you to enhance the joy in your life. There are lots of uses of these essential oils, such as you can increase your joy and happiness of your party by diffusing few oils. You can also memorize the days of winter holidays by using Cinnamon, Ginger, and a little Orange essential oil. Put a few drops of these oils in the evaporator to increase the happiness. The blend of various oils will be a unique way to enhance your mood. Some blends of essential oils help women to stabilize their hormones. The blend will only help women without affecting the hormonal balance of another person in the house. Following are some essential oils that will help you to increase your happiness.

Bergamot Essential Oil

The fresh, citrus oil and refreshing scent of the essential oils can uplift your mood. The aroma of this oil will help you to feel bright, happy and energized. It is excellent for your healthy skin and improve good health. It is useful for its antiseptic properties, particularly for the skin that is prone to acne. It is useful for eczema and other conditions that can increase stress.

Geranium Essential Oil

This is an excellent essential oil to harmonize, comfort, calm and balance your mood. It can uplift your mood and strengthen your mind to get rid of tensions and anxiety. It is a wonderful oil for skin care and treat menopause condition as well. The oil is equally good to use for a healthy and excellent skin. If you have dry and oily skin, you can use it because of its antiseptic and anti-inflammatory properties. It can heal the reasons of tension and uplift your mood.

Enhance Happiness

Wild orange: 2 drops

Wintergreen oil: 2 drops

Boost Your Mood

Wild orange oil: 2 drops

Frankincense oil: 2 drops

Cinnamon oil: 2 drops

Chillout Essential Oil

Vetiver essential oil: 2 drops

Cedarwood essential oil: 2 drops

Happy Diffuser Oil

Wild orange: 2 drops

White fir: 2 drops

Wintergreen: 1 drop

Chapter 4 – Essential Oil Diffusers to Manage Anger

There are lots of essential oils that can help you to relax. The strong aroma of these oils will relax your nerves and help you to control negative emotions. Following are some essential oils that are really beneficial for your health:

Peace and Calming Blend

You can prepare a blend of orange, tangerine, ylang-ylang, blue tansy and patchouli because this blend is excellent to manage your anger. It can promote the feelings of peace and reduce your stress level.

Directions:

If you want to treat your anger, then you should consider this blend because the massage of this oil will help you to manage anger. Use it in a diffused state and promote peace and calmness. Add a drop of oil in your bath water, or you can use it as a perfume as well.

Ylang Ylang

It is an excellent essential oil used in a diffused form to treat anger. The properties of this special essential oil will help you to reduce anxiety, blood pressure, frustration and much more.

Directions:

If you want to take the benefits of this essential oil, then apply it on your feet in a diffused form. You can also rub it on your spin on your lower back to get rid of anger.

Roman Chamomile Essential Oil

If an angry outburst is an important part of your conversation, then you should try this essential oil. This oil has magical properties to treat allergy, cleanse your blood, calm your sorrow and grieves.

Directions:

You can apply this essential oil on your throat in a diffused form. It will help you to stabilize your anger and bring your emotions to a balance.

Lavender Essential Oil

The lavender is famous for its soothing and calming properties because after its application, you can feel relaxed. It can treat allergies, digestion problems; reduce nausea and many other problems. Its regular massage will promote your good health and enhance your mood.

Directions:

The lavender can be inhaled from the bottle, or you can rub the back of your neck after taking this oil on your hands. It will help you to reduce stress and tension. The oil has excellent properties to diffuse your anger.

Geranium Essential Oil

This is an excellent essential oil, and you should include it in your daily routine. The essential oil is excellent to make your skin beautiful and support your circulatory and nervous system. It is excellent to invigorate your body tissues.

Directions:

You can use this oil to promote brain health, and it is quite easy to use because it is good to inhale it directly. Few drops of diffused geranium essential oil can be rubbed on your neck to get rid of anger.

Sandalwood Essential Oil

The sandalwood essential oil can treat your emotional issues, relieve stress and unwind the tensions. Aloes are its other name, and you can rub your backbone, wrist, and neck with the help of diffused sandalwood essential oil. This oil is really good for your skin. After its frequent use, you can be able to get rid of all tensions and anger emotions.

Blue Tansy Essential Oil

It has slightly sweet aroma and used to manage anger. If you are suffering from anger and other negative emotions, then use this essential oil because it has lots of benefits. The famous species of tansy plants are Moroccan and Chamomile.

Directions:

- Take a few drops of diffused essential oil, and apply it on your feet. It can calm your mind and alleviate the negative emotions.

- You can also add a few drops in your bath to promote the feelings of relaxation.

Soothing Blends:

Following are some blends that will help you to promote the feelings of relaxation and enhance your mood:

Blend 01:

- 1 drop Rose

- 3 drops Orange

- 1 drop Vetiver

Mix all these essential oils and pour it in the water before taking a bath. It will help you to reduce anger.

Blend 02:

- 3 drops Bergamot

- 1 drop Ylang Ylang

- 1 drop Jasmine

Add this blend to your bath water and take a bath with it to gradually reduce your anger.

Blend 03:

- 1 drop Roman Chamomile

- 2 drops Bergamot

- 2 Drops Orange Essential Oil

Take a relaxing bath after adding this blend in a bucket of water, and get the benefits of this bath.

Blend 04:

- 3 drops of Orange Essential Oil

- 2 drops of Patchouli Oil

This will be the relaxing blend for to manage your anger. Include it in a bucket of water to take a bath or add it in a diffuser to keep it in your room

Tips to Diffuse Your Blend

You can increase the amount of blend by adding your oil in a dark colored bottle made of glass and then roll the bottle between your hands. You can add a diffuser like olive oil to diffuse the blend and use this blend in your bath water.

Carrier Oils

The carrier oils are often used as a diffuser to diffuse the intensity of carrier oils. You can mix these oils with essential oils to take aromatherapy. Following are some famous and frequently used carrier oils:

- Sweet almond oil

- Olive oil

- Sunflower oil

In short, the seed, vegetable, and nut oils can be used to dilute the concentrated essential oils.

Rose Essential Oils

The rose essential oils are famous for its properties because it can be used as an antidepressant, antiseptic, antispasmodic, hepatic, uterine, stomachic, etc. The rose essential oil works well to alleviate stress, mental tension, depression, nervous ailments and various other problems. If you want to get rid of anger and mental stress, then use rose essential oil to manage this situation.

Palo Santo Essential Oil

The palo santo essential oil is used to manage anger because its scent can keep your mind free from worries and tensions. Its anti-inflammatory properties can help you to avoid cancer as well. The regular use of this oil will help you to manage anger and stress.

Diffuser

- 5 drops Cedarwood Atlas
- 4 drops Palo Santo
- 1 drop Patchouli
- 5 drops of Bergamot

Bug Repellent Diffuser of Essential Oil

Lemongrass oil: 1 drop

Thyme oil: 1 drop

Eucalyptus oil: 1 drop

Basil oil: 1 drop

Chapter 5 – Increase Your Confidence with Essential Oil Diffusers

There are lots of essential oils that are used during performing religious traditions. The exotic fragrance and purities of the essential oil can improve your mood. There are a number of essential oils that can be used to increase self-confidence.

Cypress Essential Oil

The cypress essential oil is famous for its properties because it can help you to treat lots of problems. It can help you to extricate stuck emotions. If you are feeling any tension and want to ignore everything, then push things aside and shove negative emotions. The negative emotions make it really hard to feel relaxed and the cypress can help you to bring an accurate balance to your mind and spirit. You can get rid of fear and treat your negative emotions with the help of cypress essential oil.

Directions:

You can use it in diluted form and then massage several locations of your body. You should consider the vita flex points to get optimum benefits.

Peppermint Essential Oils

If you want to enhance your energy and confidence, then the peppermint essential oil will be an excellent drug for you. There is no need to drink caffeine because the essential oil can increase your energy levels. The peppermint oil trickles the freshness and improves your mental health. It can keep you alert and enables you to tackle each task in a better way.

Directions:

Peppermint essential oil can uplift your mood and confidence. You can include a few drops of peppermint oil in your bath water to keep your mind fresh. It will reduce tension, anxiety and enhance the feelings of calmness. In the absence of tension and anxiety, you can perform in a better way.

Sandalwood Essential Oil

If you have dry or irritated skin, then you may feel low in the public places because a smooth and beautiful skin can boost your confidence. With dull and dry skin, you will only think about the negative views of people about you. If you want a glowing and healthy skin, then you should add a few drops of sandalwood essential oil in your body lotion. It will make your skin healthy and increase its glow. When you feel good in your own skin, your self-confidence will be at a higher level.

Bergamot Essential Oil

The bergamot essential oil is an excellent addition to your daily routine because it can improve the health of your skin. It is often used in the production of perfumes and has amazing healing powers. This oil is equally good for your brain because it can cure your stress, tension, and anger in a better way. If you want to increase your self-confidence, you should reduce your stress, anxiety, and tension. The Bergamot essential oil will play an important role in this.

Rosemary Essential Oil

If you want to boost your confidence, then you should focus on your personal improvement. The rosemary essential oil will increase the shine and smooth texture of your hair. Just add five drops of rosemary oil in the bottle of shampoo. It will make your hair silky and keep your scalp free from dandruff. If you are suffering from migraines, then instead of using tablets, try this oil. Use a drop of this oil and massage on your wrists. Take q few deep breaths and feel the calm sensation.

Tea Tree Essential Oil

If you are feeling any problem just because of virus and bacteria around you, then you should use tea tree oil. The oil will serve as a body bouncer and improve the immune system of your body in a natural way. It will save your money because after using this, there is no need to use expensive treatments. You can pamper your skin with the help of this oil because it may reduce the acne from your skin. Tea tree oil will be an ultimate solution of your all problems. Take a bath by adding a few drops of tea tree essential oils in water.

Chamomile Essential Oil

It is quite surprising to know that the chamomile is an excellent mood booster. If you are feeling burdened and want to get rid of these feelings, then use this oil. Just add a few drops of chamomile oil in the boiling water, and take a bath to see its magic.

Ylang-Ylang Essential Oil

If you have ylang-ylang essential oil, then you can turn your own bathroom into a spa by adding a few drops of this oil in water. This will help you to control your emotions, and you may feel relaxed. This essential oil is available in a small bottle, and you can use it in different ways. If you don't want to take a bath, then you can add a few drops in a very small bottle and spray this water on your face. It will enhance the feelings of calmness and relaxation. This is an excellent mood booster and increases your self-confidence as well.

There are lots of powerful essential oils that can increase your self-confidence and enhance your mood. You can inhale these oils or take a bath by adding a few drops. If you want to enjoy enough benefits of essential oils, then find the right oil for you to restore your energy. It will increase your self-confidence by boosting your mood.

Diffuser to Increase Your Alertness

Wild orange oil: 2 drops

Peppermint oil: 2 drops

Fresh Diffuser of Essential Oil

Lavender oil: 2 drops

Lemon oil: 2 drops

Rosemary oil: 2 drops

Odor Eliminator

Lemon oil: 2 drops

Melaleuca oil: 1 drop

Cilantro oil: 1 drop

Lime oil: 1 drop

Seasonal Diffuser

Lavender oil: 2 drops

Lemon oil: 2 drops

Peppermint oil: 2 drops

Citrus Explosion Oil

Lemon oil: 1 drop

Wild orange oil: 2 drops

Lime oil: 1 drop

Grapefruit oil: 1 drop

Deep Breath Essential Oil Diffusers

Bergamot oil: 1 drop

Patchouli oil: 1 drop

Ylang ylang oil: 1 drop

Respiratory Blend

Lemon oil: 1 drop

Eucalyptus oil: 1 drop

Peppermint oil: 2 drops

Rosemary oil: 1 drop

Flower Garden Diffuser

Lavender oil: 2 drops

Geranium oil: 1 drop

Roman Chamomile oil: 2 drops

Precautionary Tips for Essential Oil

It is really good to use essential oils, but you have to consider safety and effectiveness. Following are some general guideline and precautions that will help you:

- You need to keep essential oils away from the reach of children and pets.

- The essential oils with high menthol like peppermint should not be used on the throat and neck of the children under 30 months.

- The essential oils can't dilute in the water; therefore, you can mix them in the vegetable oil to dissolve in water.

- The oils are available in the concentrated state; therefore, you should use them in diluted form. The concentrated oil should not come in contact with the sensitive skin areas.

- Undiluted oils should not be directly poured into the bath water.

- If you have sensitive skin, then the oil should not be applied directly on the skin. Dilute it with a carrier oil and then apply to the neat and clean soles of the feet.

- If you have allergies, then you should be careful while using essential oils. The sole of your feet is the least sensitive area, and you can apply oil on the sole.

- Some essential oils have strong caustic properties; dilute these essential oils before using them.

- Some citrus essential like orange, lemon and bergamot and petitgrain should not be applied directly on the skin if you have to go out. These oils are phototoxic and you need to avoid direct sunlight for almost 48hours.

- Before trying any kind of essential oil, you need to do a patch test of the diluted oil to know if it is irritating you.

- A number of essential oils are not good to ingest; therefore, you have to be careful. Properly know the properties of the essential oils before ingesting them. It is good to take the advice of your health care advisor before consuming any oil.

- If you have sensitive skin, heart and kidney problems, asthma, and other serious medical conditions, then you should consult your doctor for the safety of any essential oil for you.

- The properties of essential oil can't be judged on the basis of the properties of its plants.

- Keep the essential oils away from heat, flame, and all ignition sources.

- You need to be careful while applying essential oils on the skin because some personal care products may contain synthetic and petrochemicals. These can penetrate and remain in the skin and fatty tissues for various days. The essential oils can react with these chemicals to cause irritation, nausea, and other displeasures.

- There can be a strong reaction of essential oils on the body because of the chemicals in food, water, and the environment. If your skin gets any reaction, then stop the use of essential oil and start internal cleansing before resuming to the regular routine. You can increase the water intake to reduce any adverse reaction.

Precautions for An Accident with Essential Oils

If an essential oil falls into your eyes accidentally, the immediately flush it with cold milk or vegetable oil to dilute the oil. If you still feel any stinging, you can consult a doctor immediately.

You can use cream or vegetable oil to remove the additional essential oils from your skin. Use soap and warm water to remove additional oil from the skin.

If you ingest any essential oil accidently, then you can call national poison control center for assistance.

Conclusion

Essential oils can affect your mind and emotions in a better way because of their strong scent. The aromas of essential oils can have a good impact on your emotions, and can reach deep into the psyche. It can keep your mind relaxed and uplift your spirit. You will be amazed to know that the smelling sense of human beings is 10,000 times more sensitive than other senses.

The scents can travel at a faster rate to the brain and improve your sound and sight at the same time. It is better to use essential oils for your emotions as compared to medicines. There are lots of side effects directly linked to the medications, but the essential oils have no side-effects.

The essential oils work in a particular way because whenever you inhale an essential oil, the molecules of its odor may travel up to the nose allied to the nerves of the olfactory membranes in the nose. These molecules can excite the inside layer of nerve cells and enhance the electrical impulses to the olfactory bulb of your brain. This particular part of your brain transmits the impulses to the amygdala. The amygdala is the place where the memories are usually stored, and connected to the limbic system of the brain.

FREE Bonus Reminder

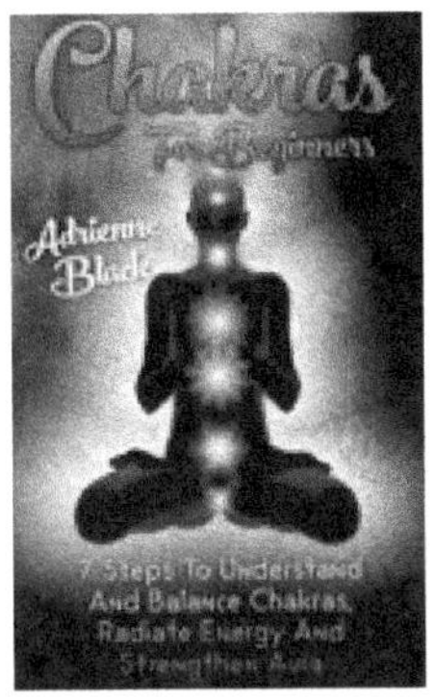

If you have not grabbed it yet, please go ahead and download your special bonus E book *"Chakras for Beginners. 7 Steps To Understand And Balance Chakras, Radiate Energy, And Strengthen Aura"*.

Simply Click the Button Below

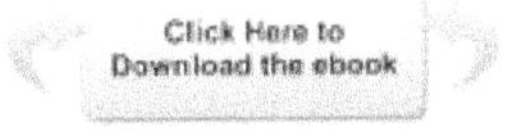

OR **Go to This Page**

http://lifehacksworld.com/free

BONUS #2: More Free & Discounted Books

Do you want to receive more Free & Discounted Books?

We have a mailing list where we send out our new Books when they go free or with a discount on Kindle. Click on the link below to sign up for Free & Discount Book Promotions.

=> Sign Up for Free & Discount Book Promotions <=

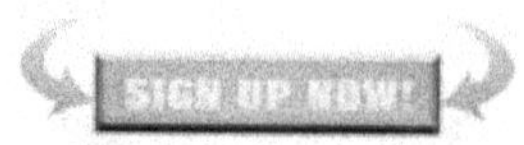

OR Go to this URL

http://zbit.ly/1WBb1Ek